Healthy Living:

How to Purify Your Body in a Polluted World

(Healthy Living Book)

Gina 'The Veggie Goddess' Matthews

Copyright

Disclaimer:

All contents of this book are strictly for educational and informational purposes only. The author and publisher will not be held liable for any use or misuse of any information contained or mentioned within this book. The author is not a doctor, and none of the information contained within this book, is meant to replace or displace the guidance of one's personal doctor. The author strongly advises that everyone always be under the care of a qualified health care practitioner, and seek the advise and instruction from their health care provider, before making any changes to their health care practices.

TABLE OF CONTENTS

INTRODUCTION

What does healthy living mean? For me, health living means embracing a lifestyle of clean eating and life habits, including the reduction and elimination of toxic elements from one's diet, body care, and home care practices. Of course, it is much more detailed than that, but, at the same time, it really is as simple as that.

In a span of half of a generation, we as a society have gone from living a fairly natural lifestyle, to one that is inundated with chemicals and toxins in every conceivable form. In the average family's home, all you have to do is read the label on any of the food products in their pantry or fridge, or, any label on their collection of personal care and home care products, and you will see a plethora of words you can't pronounce, or even know what they mean on those labels. The average family uses toxic lab-made products at unprecedented levels, yet they are surprised that their family's health and well-being, is anything but healthy or well.

The human body is quite adaptable to change, yet, one thing it cannot do is thrive and survive, with regular exposure and ingestion of chemicals and toxins. The human body has a web of detection and elimination processes that signal the exposure or consumption of a toxin, and, it goes to work immediately trying to rid the offending toxin(s) from your body. If one continues on to regularly expose and consume these toxic elements, especially without regular detoxification practices, the body resorts to other measures in an attempt to keep you alive. This includes weight gain that you can't lose (there is a reason why), skin eruptions, bouts of sickness, illness, disease, and then the eventual demise of a functioning body. What the body is doing, is attempting to purge these chemicals and toxins from your body, any way that it can. When these attempts to detoxify the body are constantly being ignored, and overriden by continuous unhealthy living habits, the effects become compounded and more severe. Contrary to marketing ploys by many consumer products, chemicals are not safe for human exposure or consumption, even in diluted form. Just because something doesn't harm or kill you immediately, doesn't mean it won't eventually.

For far too long now, the corrupt practices of the FDA, USDA, EPA, and other so-called consumer protection agencies, have allowed the continuous influx of chemicals and toxins into our food, personal care, and home care product supply. Furthermore, the manufacturers of these products use downright misleading and false marketing tactics to promote their poisonous products to the consumer. Why? For money, money, and more money. It starts with the initial profits from the sales of their products, but then continues on when the people using and consuming them become riddled with illness and disease. There is big profit to be had in the world of sickness. The 'cut it' and 'drug it' mentality of the western world's medical system rakes in trillions of dollars every year. And, anything that threatens those 'cut it' and 'drug it' profits, is met with threats of retaliation. (That in itself is a story and book for another time.) Natural and alternative health care practices and practitioners are ridiculed and demeaned, typically through the use of more misleading and falsified marketing tactics.

In addition to being a vegetarian and vegan blogger and author, I am also a holistic therapist by trade. I provide a multitude of Asian-based holistic therapies to my clientele, as well as educate and guide them on healthy eating and healthy living habits. I spent my younger years, as a paramedic with the fire department, a 911 dispatcher and a MA (medical assistant) in the cardiothoracic surgery department of Mayo hospital. That being mentioned let me get this out of the way. When it comes to emergency care, acute care, and some specialty care, there is no other country that I would rather be, than the United States, to get the emergency, acute, or specialty care medical attention that I might be in need of. The United States has superior medical facilities, health practitioners and diagnostic equipment and testing to serve those needs. However, when it comes to definitive care, I personally feel that the medical care system is severely sub-par, and even abusive. Natural health and well-being is not on the agenda of the definitive health care system. Selling unnecessary surgery and drugs is, both of which, is far too often the 'go-to' solution when one goes to pay their doctor a visit.

I am impassioned with natural health, and all the healthy living habits that that encompasses. I practice what I teach, and, at just shy of 50 years old, I look and feel decades younger than my chronological age, I am free of any ill health, and very rarely ever get sick. I truly love teaching what I know to others, and will soon be closing my clientele practice, so that I may write and teach on the subjects of vegetarian, vegan, and raw nutrition, as well as natural health and holistic healing on a full-time basis.

Detoxification and cleansing practices, is one of those many subject matters within the scope of natural health and holistic healing, and of course, the topic of this book. Anyone who is aligned with healthy and natural living should be regularly including detoxification methods into their lifestyle, as well as clean living habits. While that may sound daunting to those who might be just now making a commitment to living a healthier life, it really isn't. Cleaning up your body and life is not a race, so you should never feel like it's an all-or-nothing approach. Do what you can, as you can, and celebrate those little successes along the way. One of the most common breakpoints of doing the all-or-nothing approach, to detoxifying and cleansing, is that if you try to do a complete overhaul all at once, you will typically view any misstep as a complete system failure, and then just give up. Avoid this all-too-common mistake that many people make, and tailor your detoxification efforts to your specific lifestyle and needs. It's ok to start slow, but, be careful to not use that as an excuse to stall, or have huge time gaps in-between your detoxification efforts.

So, celebrate your commitment, or re-commitment, to healthy living, and let's dive in on how you can detoxify and cleanse your body and living environment, in easy-to-do steps that will bring you into better health and well-being, starting today.

Gina 'The Veggie Goddess' Matthews

PART I:
COMING CLEAN – LET'S DETOXIFY

CHAPTER 1 – HOW WE BECOME TOXIC

You hear the words detox and cleansing being thrown around all the time in the natural health arena, but, for many people, they really aren't quite sure what detoxing and cleansing really entails. In this comprehensive book, we are going to cover precisely what it means to "detox", what the "cleansing crisis" is, and varies ways (both gently and more aggressively) we can assist our bodies in this full-body detoxification and cleansing process.

By using a variety of drugless, natural detoxification methods, which I will outline in detail throughout this book, harmful stored toxins and wastes can then be extracted and eliminated from the body. Providing a clean internal environment within the body is vital in order to facilitate the necessary upkeep of cellular repair and rebuilding processes within and throughout the body. Additionally, a clean healthy body environment is also vitally important for supporting and enabling the immune system to be able to prevent and overcome harmful and deteriorating conditions from taking hold with the body, which would otherwise result in chronic illness and disease.

What is Detoxification?

Detoxification is something our bodies are designed to do both naturally, and, every single day. It's one of the most basic and automatic functions of our body. Detoxification is the normal body process of eliminating or neutralizing toxins through the colon, liver, kidneys, lymph and skin. And, just as our heart beats non-stop and our lungs breathe non-stop, so too are our metabolic processes, which are at work continuously disposing of accumulated wastes and toxic matter. Our bodies must flush out these toxins in order to survive and function properly, and our bodies accomplish this by sweating out toxins, breathing out toxins, filtering and neutralizing toxins via our kidneys and liver, and excreting them via our urine and bowel movements. If our bodies didn't have the ability to remove these toxins, we would die rather quickly. And, in today's world, the effects of accumulated toxins being stored within the body 'show up' in the form of many imbalances and disease, such as obesity, skin disorders, digestive disorders, mental decline, fertility issues, endocrine imbalances, and on and on.

Why We Need To Detox

Western societies are exposed to chemicals and pollutants on an unprecedented scale, and we are presented with the daunting challenge of trying to make amends with Mother Earth, and purify and clean our environment from the mess we made of it. We can, should, and hopefully will make it better. But, even if there was a sudden and complete ban on all toxic chemicals and pollutants, the residues of the mountainous accumulation of environmental poisons and toxins is so great, that it would take centuries to potentially correct and bring our environment back into natural balance.

Since we cannot completely remove toxins from our environment, nor can we completely avoid them in our everyday life, we must learn to do our best to avoid and minimize self-toxification, make sensible and healthier lifestyle choices, and use regular detoxification methods to keep our bodies and living spaces clean and free from toxic debris as much as possible. By including regular detoxification methods into your lifestyle, you will not only purge recent harmful substances from your body, you will also assist in the elimination of the accumulated toxins and waste products that our stored deep within your body tissues.

Where Do These Toxins Come From?

We our quite literally surrounded and bombarded with toxins and poisons in our everyday life.

Industrial chemicals pollute our water through run-offs; pesticides and additives are added to virtually all commercially prepared foods; heavy metals; anesthetics; drugs (both prescribed and street drugs); environmental hormones; the potent chemicals used in commercial household cleaning products, building products, grooming products, and outdoor yard and garden products. Every single body system and every single body tissue is affected by these toxins, and the effects range from mild skin irritation, to harmful health conditions, to the inability to lose weight, and all the way up to actual DNA alteration.

Preservatives and Pesticides

Preservatives are poisons added to foods to prevent oxidation and to kill and inhibit the growth of microorganisms. This enables a longer shelf-life and a lot more money to food manufacturers. This also has adversely affected the lively-hood of local farmers, who are a dying breed. Sulfites are just one of the commonly used food preservatives used in many processed foods, beverages and drugs. Sulfites cause a long list of disturbances in the body, and some can be quite severe and even fatal to some. They are especially troublesome for asthmatics. So harmful in fact, that the U.S. banned the use of sulfites in restaurant salad bars. Numerous other chemical preservatives and food additives are commonly used in commercially prepared foods, and all have serious health consequences. These include "flavors", flavor enhancers, "spices", color enhancers, emulsifiers, sweeteners, monosodium glutamate (under any one of its cleverly disguised names), and so on.

Pesticides are another common contaminant, which are intentionally and continuously added to our environment. Pesticides are known to cause birth defects, sterility, learning disorders, tumors, organ damage, central nervous system impairment and more. We cannot usually see or taste pesticides in our food, so it is often impossible to detect them. Unless you are eating organic produce, and, organic meats if you are a carnivore, you can be sure you are eating a whopping daily dose of pesticides with your commercially processed produce and meats. And, even more disturbing, is that the FDA, USDA and other government agencies are contributing to this problem. These agencies have actually regulated unprecedented tolerances for pesticide residues in foods.

Pesticides are not only a contaminant of produce, but in animal products as well. Pesticide residues concentrate in fat tissues, and fat tissues intermingle with muscle fibers. This means that every time you consume commercially processed meats, you are also consuming pesticide residues, hormone and drug residues, and any disease residues contained in that animal's tissues.

"Incidental food contaminants" are substances that find their way into food as a result of some phase of harvesting, processing, storage or packaging.

Examples include: animal hairs, rat droppings, tiny bits of plastic, glass, paper, tin, and other substances, as well as chemicals such as solvents used in the processing phase. The government considers the migration of "incidental food additives" to be unavoidable and allows certain measurable amounts of these substances into foods. For example, each 3.5 ounce can of mushrooms is allowed to contain up to 19 maggots and 74 mites. And, each can of tomato paste or pizza sauce is allowed to contain 30 or more fly eggs per 100 grams. In fact, the average person consumes 2 pounds of flies, maggots and mites every year in their commercially prepared food products, without even knowing it.

The use of common household cleaning products and grooming products is another serious health hazard, all in itself. Remember, just because your favorite household product is manufactured by "the family company", doesn't mean it is family safe or family friendly.

Now that we have expanded on the specific ways in which our bodies are continuously exposed to and accumulating harmful toxins, hopefully, so too has your awareness of the need to assist your body in the removal of these harmful toxins through regular and natural detoxification methods. As we move onto the next chapter, we will cover what exactly that means, what to expect, and how to make your detoxification and cleansing efforts a more tolerable and pleasant experience.

CHAPTER 2 – UNDERSTANDING THE HEALING CRISIS

When you embark on a detoxification or cleansing method, chances are, you will experience some degree of physical and/or mental discomfort at some point during the process. The discomfort you experience is what is referred to as "The Healing Crisis". In fact, sickness is a form of healing crisis. Your body develops a cold, flu or fever, for example, in an attempt to throw off a virus, or some other harmful invader. During this time of sickness, you will feel worse before you feel better. This time of feeling worse, is your "healing crisis". When you understand this, you will not be so alarmed when you experience times of feeling worse, before you feel better. In fact, this is a clear sign that your body is successfully ridding itself of stored toxins and waste products, and repairing and rebuilding itself. Additionally, when you understand this, you will also not blame your detoxification efforts for making you feel worse, or say that the detox method must not be working. This is the number one reason why so many people shy away from detoxification and cleansing. They don't understand why they feel worse, and / or they just don't want to ride-out that time of discomfort before feeling better.

What you must realize is that as all those long-stored, accumulated layers of toxins are being pulled out of your cellular spaces, it is flooding your bloodstream and lymph system with waste products. While those waste products are circulating in your bloodstream and other excretory pathways, and making their way out of your system, you body will feel less than optimal. Once your body has started to flush out these long-stored toxins and waste products, and the healing crisis subsides, you will be amazed at how much better you will feel, both in body and mind.

Examples of Getting Worse Before Getting Better

During detoxification, your body is continuously pulling out numerous toxins and harmful substances from their embedded cellular spaces. Your body may produce a fever. A fever's purpose is to thin the lymph, and helps your lymph system do its job, which is to contain and purge harmful substances from the body. When your lymph is too thick and stagnant, it can't do this efficiently. This is especially the case for those who do not exercise regularly, for our lymph system has no pump, and it is only through physical movement that we manually 'pump' our lymph through our bodies. We can also produce an "artificial fever" by means of sauna therapy, bath therapy and exercising. Viruses can't survive when body temperature is elevated, which is why our body develops a fever in response to one. Elevated body temperature also spurs our immune system as well. So, as you can see, a fever is nature's way of detoxifying and cleansing our body of harmful invaders.

Other examples of getting worse before getting better, and how our bodies intelligently know and react to toxins, is to produce other various symptoms of sickness such as a runny nose; diarrhea, nausea, sneezing, coughing, lose of appetite, fatigue, etc. Our bodies are much smarter than we are, and intuitively know how to help us heal and balance our health. When we experience sneezing, coughing and a runny nose, this is our body producing mucus so that the invading toxins can be contained and eliminated when we cough, sneeze or blow our nose. Vomiting and diarrhea is our body eliminating toxins via our digestive system. Loss of appetite and fatigue is our body's way of slowing down and conserving energy that needs to be directed towards the healing and repair process, instead of digesting heavy meals. Pain is our body's way of signally a body part that needs attention.

Support Don't Suppress the Healing Crisis

One of the most counter-productive things we can do when we are experiencing any of the above bodily effects, is to suffocate or suppress any uncomfortable symptoms, by taking over-the-counter medications. Stifling symptoms with over-the-counter medications, prevents the exiting of the offending toxins and microbes, and in fact, it pushes them deeper into our body tissues. As a general rule, our bodies will create 3 attempts of eradicating a cycle of toxins, harmful substances, or imbalance from our body by a specific means, such as a fever, cold, diarrhea, fatigue, pain, skin eruptions, etc. If we keep suppressing these attempts, the body has no choice but to come up with more intense and more uncomfortable ways to evacuate these toxins and poisons. And so, that cold now becomes bronchitis or pneumonia. That diarrhea now advances to irritable bowel or colitis. Those minor skin eruptions are now eczema or psoriasis. Those periodic bouts of fatigue now become full-blown chronic fatigue syndrome. If you are continuously experiencing these types of health disturbances, try looking backwards to see how many times your body tried to give you warning signs.

It is far better to support your body during a time of healing crisis vs. suppressing the uncomfortable symptoms. Supporting your body means taking extra rest and extra water. It means eating light, nature-made foods and eliminating caffeine, alcohol and any unnecessary drugs. If you have a fever, it means drinking plenty of cool water and keeping the head cool, while allowing the body to sweat out the offending toxins and poisons.

If you have a runny nose or are sneezing frequently, don't suppress it with drugs, blow your nose and get those toxins out. If you have a cough, ease the soreness and hacking with warm tea or water and taking some spoonfuls of raw honey throughout the day. Raw honey naturally suppresses a cough, while soothing and healing the throat. It also means avoiding all cold foods and beverages, which can instigate a coughing attack.

If you are experiencing diarrhea or vomiting, allow your body to expel those toxins. Your body is going through a lot of processes, to eliminate these toxins from either end of your digestive system. Think about it for a minute. Why in the world would you want to hold onto your s$#*? In the case of either diarrhea or vomiting, you want to make absolutely sure to drink enough water to replace those fluids you are losing. And, add a pinch of real mineralized sea salt to every other glass of filtered water you drink, to help your body replace lost electrolytes as well.

Suppressing your healing crisis with drugs, only serves to also suppress the elimination of the toxins and harmful substances from your body. If these toxins can't come out, or aren't allowed to come out, then they retreat deeper and deeper within your cellular tissues, only to resurface later, with more pronounced discomfort and more pronounced harm to your health and well-being. If these toxins are not able or allowed to be flushed from your system, your body's secondary response in protecting you from toxic overload, is to direct and store these toxins deep within your fat cells. Why the fat cells? Because, your body would become so overloaded with toxins and poisons if these wastes were allowed to circulate and settle into your organs, and other vital areas, that you would quite literally die from toxic shock. That is why for many people, no matter how much they exercise or eat right, they can't seem to lose those last 10-20 pounds. It is commonly due to the toxic load they have stored in their body tissues. Detoxification and cleansing will help rid the body of these accumulated toxins, and allow the body to release any stubborn excess weight (which was protecting us and keeping us alive - literally), and function at more optimal levels.

Slow and Steady or Fast and Furious

When undergoing any detoxification or cleansing method or program, please keep the following in mind. If you experience frequent sickness or have a lot of health issues, then you'll want to go slow and steady with your detoxification efforts. The reason why is, that you will be releasing and dumping a lot of toxins into your body's excretory pathways for elimination, and you don't want to overwhelm your already compromised body and health. So, the sicker or weaker you are, or if you have a multitude of health issues going on, take things slow. If you are of relatively good health and shape, you can typically go a bit more aggressively with your detoxification efforts. This can mean employing them more often, or for a longer period of time, or undergoing several detoxification methods at the same time.

In either case, always pay close attention to your body. Listen to the signals it is giving you. If you feel you are being overwhelmed by any particular detoxification method, then don't do it as often, or long. Or, you can try a different, gentler alternative. And, as much as you possibly can, don't suppress your healing crisis. Support your healing, and ride out the uncomfortable symptoms. They will subside. If you're going to undergo a detoxification and cleansing method, only to suppress the healing crisis with aspirin, anti-cough, anti-sneeze, and anti-ache medication, then you may as well just skip the whole process all-together, because you will void out most, if not all, of the cleansing and healing benefits.

CHAPTER 3 – HEAT THERAPIES FOR DETOXIFICATION

In the past, an artificial fever was almost always induced to treat a person suffering from an infectious condition. It was common knowledge, that increasing a patient's temperature to the point of inducing profuse sweating would "sweat the infection out". And, it works for both viral and bacterial infections, as well as many other conditions.

Nowadays, fever is often mistakenly thought of as an undesirable symptom of illness, because it increases our discomfort during this time. Because of this, people will often readily take medication to reduce their fever, instead of supporting the process by drinking cool water, taking cool baths, eliminating all heavy foods and getting plenty of rest. This is often a great mistake, as this tends to stifle the natural detoxification and healing process and prolongs the duration of illness, as well as migrates the harmful virus or bacteria back deep within the body tissues. Elevating internal body temperature is one of the body's built-in major defenses against invading organisms. It is vital to the healing process for many illnesses and imbalances, because bacteria and viruses, which cause most illnesses as well as other toxic imbalances in the body, are heat sensitive.

Examples of some of the conditions that respond to heat therapy ("artificially induced fever") are: influenza (flu), upper and lower respiratory tract infections, bladder problems, urinary tract infections, chickenpox, shingles, herpes, syphilis, gonorrhea and even AIDS. Virtually every known disease-causing virus and bacteria is vulnerable to heat, and medical literature is chock-full of such references to the use of heat therapy.

The Ultimate Detoxifier

Heat therapy (natural, or induced) stimulates all organs and glands, including the immune system, to neutralize and cleanse toxins from the body. Heat therapy also stimulates the production rate of white blood cells, which increase the generation and circulation of antibodies and interferon (a protein that attacks viruses and also has potent cancer-fighting properties). The increased number of white blood cells boosts the immune systems capability to combat invading microorganisms and remove toxic debris.

The body stores most toxins in fatty tissues. Heat therapy is one of the best ways to pull embedded toxins out of the fat cells, and eliminate them from the body. Toxins are removed through all the organs of elimination: skin, bowels and kidneys. Heat therapy also cleanses clogged skin pores and removes uric acid, heavy metals and metabolic wastes from the body. In fact, 30% of all toxic body wastes are eliminated through perspiration alone!

Heat Therapies

You can induce an "artificial fever" by many various methods such as: soaking in a tub of hot water; sitting in a sauna; moderate exercise (especially outdoors); and even through the use of hot water bottles and blankets. I will briefly touch on each of these methods below, and encourage you to choose a method that works best for you. <u>A word of caution</u>: Do NOT use electrical heat sources, such as electric blankets, pads or heaters. These devices emit electromagnetic radiation that disrupts the healing process.

Strive for 15-30 minutes per session if you can, but again, always listen to your body. If you can only tolerate 5 or 10 minutes, then only do 5 or 10 minutes. This is not a contest, so go at the pace your body is telling you to go, and extend your time gradually. Heat therapy may cause you to feel exhausted and weak, just as if you had a vigorous workout, because the cells and tissues of the body have in effect, been working at an accelerated rate. For this reason, I usually recommended that heat therapy be used prior to going to bed, as much as possible. You will sleep like a baby, and when you are in a state of restful deep sleep, your body is better able to eliminate toxic waste. If you find that you don't feel tired after a heat therapy session, this may be a sign that you didn't do it long enough, and you may wish to add a few minutes to your next heat therapy session.

Hot Bath - Probably the most convenient heat therapy source is a bathtub full of hot water. To be effective, you need to be completely submerged, except for your head, and in water that is hot enough to raise your own body temperature. As the water cools, drain some out and replace with more hot water, keeping the temperature as hot as you can comfortably tolerate. Keep a cold wash cloth next to the tub, and place on the back of your neck as needed, to keep your head cool. Ideally, you want to remain in the bath for 30 minutes, but even as little as 10 minutes is beneficially. Helpful Hint: If your tub is too small to fully submerge yourself, then you can cut open a large trash bag, or purchase a cheap plastic drop cloth (easy to find at your local dollar store), and drape it over the top of you while you are in the tub, to help retain the heat in the water and in you.

Footbaths - Footbaths have a less dramatic effect on the body than a full tub bath, but they are effective nonetheless, because the soles of your feet are major portals for both absorption and elimination. And, because a footbath has a gentler effect, it is recommended for those who don't have a tub, can't get into a tub, or need to take a gentler, or slower, route with detoxification and cleansing. As with a full tub bath, make the water as hot as you can comfortably tolerate, and submerse your feet fully, and up to your calves if you have a foot tub deep enough. Stay in the footbath for 15 - 30 minutes. Even though it is a gentler means of detoxifying, it should still leave you feeling relaxed and/or tired. If it doesn't, then you need to stay in longer.

Exercise - Which type of exercise best supports detoxification? Any type of exercise that you can do comfortably without injury, that gets your whole body moving and your body fluids circulating will be beneficial. Perform your exercise long enough to induce a good sweat. To help you induce a good sweat, you can wear layers of warm, breathable clothing, but avoid wearing any constrictive clothing. Wearing tight-fitting clothing severely hampers lymph circulation, which disrupts the detoxification and cleansing process.

Sauna - There are 3 varieties of saunas: dry heat, moist heat and infrared heat saunas. If you have access to, or can afford an infrared sauna, this is by far the best sauna therapy option there is. The heat from an infrared sauna penetrates the body far deeper than dry or moist heat saunas do. And, even though infrared heat penetrates far deeper, pulling toxins from deeply imbedded cellular tissues, they don't get near as hot, which makes them much more comfortable to use, and for longer periods of time.

Hot Water Bottle Method - If you don't want to do any of the above methods, you can induce heat therapy with the hot water bottle method. Dress in warm, loose clothing, including socks, and gather several thick, warm blankets. Next, fill a couple hot water bottles with near boiling water. Get under the layer of blankets, and position your hot water bottles around your body. If possible, have someone tuck in the corners of the blankets to avoid any hot air from escaping. Try to remain under your water bottle heated blankets for 30 minutes, or as long as you can tolerate. Remember, the goal is to induce a profuse sweat, as a means for the toxins to be eliminated.

Why You Need To Shower or Wash Off After Your Heat Therapy Session

No matter which heat therapy method you chose, you will always need to conclude your therapy session with a quick shower or sponge bath. Why? You have just induced a profuse sweat, and in this sweat, is metabolic waste and toxic debris. If this toxic perspiration is not washed off, metabolic wastes and toxins can be quickly reabsorbed into the body, as well as become a breeding ground for microorganisms.

CAUTION: Pregnant women, those with high blood pressure or any existing heart conditions, those who have had a stroke or major head trauma, as well as those who currently have a fever or infection should avoid any method of heat therapy until their condition has changed.

Heat therapy as a means for regular detoxification is accessible to just about everybody, and should always be a regular part of your healthy lifestyle.

CHAPTER 4 – ADDITIONAL DETOXIFICATION METHODS

Comparing the human body to a car, detoxification methods clean out accumulated waste deposits, so you aren't running with a 'dirty engine' or driving with the brakes on, so to speak. After completing either an intensive detoxification program, or regularly using detoxification methods in your healthy lifestyle routine (ideally, you want to do both), the body starts to repair, rebalance and rebuild, and energy levels rise physically, psychologically and sexually. Creativity begins to expand, your outlook and attitude change, and, you start feeling like a different (and better) person, because you are. That's because cleansing, along with lifestyle and diet improvement, quite literally change your cellular make-up.

Let's now cover some additional detoxification methods you can be using (and is recommended) to reduce and eliminate toxic wastes from your body, helping to keep your body, mind and spirit clear, balanced and functioning at it's most optimal capacity.

Enemas - Enemas are an important part of a cleansing detox program, and are safe to use periodically, even when you're are not actively embarking on a full detoxification protocol. Enemas are especially helpful during a "healing crisis" (which I covered in Chapter 2), as it speeds up the removal of metabolic wastes, toxic wastes and drug residues from your body. Headaches, migraines and skin conditions all respond quickly to enema therapy. Enema therapy releases old, encrusted colon waste and discharges parasites. It also freshens the G.I. tract, and makes any detoxification or cleansing process easier and more thorough.

Ear Coning or Ear Candling - Ear coning is an ancient healing process used by almost every healing tradition. It is used to gently remove excess ear wax, fungus and yeast from the ear canals. It is also very stimulating to the lymph system, which then helps accelerate toxin elimination from all of our body's excretory pathways. Ear coning can also help clear itching and mold caused by candida yeast, it helps relieve pain and pressure in the ear, and aids in flushing out of any parasites that may be growing in the ear.

Skin Brushing – (I also have an entire chapter covering skin brushing in Part II of this book.) The skin is our body's largest organ, and a great deal of waste product is eliminated through our skin. The human body is constantly shedding skin cells, and if we don't help in the full removal of these sloughing dead skin tissues, our skin's pores become clogged and the removal of toxic waste debris then becomes hampered. Regular daily bathing helps us remove this layer of dead skin tissue. To further support and accelerate the rate of healthy skin cell turnover, stimulate your lymph system, and help facilitate the rapid removal of all toxic debris, you can perform a simple dry skin brushing prior to bathing or showering. You will need to use a moderately stiff brush with only natural fibers, use firm stroking motions, and always brush in the direction of your heart, which is where the lymph enters the bloodstream. NEVER skin brush over varicose veins, any skin eruptions or wounds, the face, the stomach (if pregnant) or genital area.

Hot-Cold Hydrotherapy - This technique simply involves alternating applications of hot water and cold water. Hot-cold hydrotherapy can be done in the shower, bathtub, a sitz bath, or through the use of hot and cold wraps or packs. When you subject the body to heat (hot water), the blood moves to the surface of the body, and stimulates lymph flow. When you subject the body to cold (cold water), the blood moves to the innermost areas in the body, and again, also stimulates lymph flow. The alternating of the two significantly increases circulation, lymph flow, and oxygen and nutrient distribution throughout the body, including to all your organs and glands. This is very balancing to all your body systems, and it helps regulate your digestive system, circulatory system, nervous system, and especially important, your excretory system.

When using this method in the shower, simply alternate 1 minute of hot water with 1 minute of cold water. Do this several times either at the beginning or end of your shower. To use this method in the bathtub, start out with a tub of water as hot as you can tolerate. After 10-15 minutes, drain some of the water and replace it with cold water (to tolerance), and remain submerged in the water for an additional 5 minutes or longer if you can. For sitz baths, do the same as you would the tub method, but with just enough water to cover the pelvic region. When using hot and cold wraps, alternate the application of your hot and cold pack for 5 minutes each, and make sure to place a towel between the hot or cold pack and your skin. (Do not place hot or cold packs directly against bare skin, to avoid injury.) Do this several times if you can, or to tolerance. CAUTION: Do NOT use this method if you have high blood pressure or any type of heart condition, have had a stroke or any kind of head trauma, or are pregnant.

Castor Oil Packs - Castor Oil Packs have been used for centuries, and are highly effective at stimulating and balancing one's elimination system. Castor oil packs are very cleansing to your liver, and can be used to support any detoxification method you are currently using, to aid in quicker elimination of toxins from the body. Castor Oil Packs can also be used to soften and breakup both external and internal scar tissue. CAUTION: Should NOT be used during menstruation, by pregnant women, if you have a current fever, or any type of hemorrhaging. You also need to perform a castor oil pack treatment on an empty stomach, so wait at least 2-3 hours after eating. Castor oil packs greatly relieve stagnation from the body, and stimulate the flow of lymph, blood, oxygen and nutrients, while at the same time, extricating and flushing out embedded stored toxins from cellular tissues.

Castor oil packs stain, so wear clothes you don't mind staining, and use old towels or sheets underneath you during treatment time. To do, you'll first soak a piece of flannel cloth or cheese cloth with castor oil. (You can actually purchase a complete castor oil pack kit at most health food stores.) Wring out any excess, fold and place over the body area you wish to treat. Next, cover the area with a piece of plastic, such as cling wrap, to prevent and reduce the amount of leakage and dripping of the oil. On top of the plastic, place a small towel and a hot water bottle. The heat from the hot water bottle will quickly transport the castor oil deep within the layers of body tissues. Allow the castor oil pack to remain on for 30-60 minutes. You can use this time to read, nap or meditate. This method of detoxification can be quite powerful for some, especially those with multiple or more significant health issues. You can perform a castor oil pack treatment 2-5 times a week, adjusting the duration of your treatment times and frequency based on how your body reacts. If your detoxification symptoms are too strong (the healing crisis), than simply reduce the time and frequency of treatments.

These additional detoxification methods are by no means an all-inclusive list, but they are some of the more common methods, and are of no-cost or low-cost to undergo. Try them out, and see which ones you like and which ones your body responds to most effectively. For healthier individuals, you can use several methods at one time for more intense detoxification and cleansing effects. And, for those with multiple or more serious health concerns, try them out one at a time, and give yourself several days in-between to allow your body to process and eliminate the stirred-up toxins.

Always be sure to support any detoxification method by drinking plenty of extra filtered water each and every day, and avoiding eating and drinking the very substances you are trying to cleanse your body from. You can further support your body's detoxification and cleansing efforts, by reducing stress as much as possible, getting ample sleep, and eating a light vegetarian-based diet, preferably using only organic produce.

CHAPTER 5 – CLEANSING THROUGH NUTRITION AND SUPPLEMENTS

To further support your detoxification and cleansing efforts, you ideally also want to be transitioning to a nature-made, organic foods based diet, with supplementation as needed to keep your transforming body, mind and spirit healthy, clear and balanced. You will also avoid consuming any of the toxic foods and beverages that you are trying to cleanse from your body. There is no sense in detoxifying and cleansing, if you are only going to intentionally mistreat and abuse your body afterwards with fast foods, processed foods, too much alcohol, using chemically-laden toiletries, and toxic household and garden products. If you do, your cleansing results will be short-lived. The good news is, as you continue to support your health and well-being with regular detoxification and cleansing methods, unhealthy food cravings are considerably diminished, your sleep patterns start to regulate, excess fat is eliminated and your weight starts to stabilize, and you start to effortlessly attune to healthier lifestyle habits.

Natural Foods Diet vs. Fad Diet

A natural foods diet is not a fad diet. Fad diets are usually unbalanced nutritionally, short-term, don't address better eating habits and don't eliminate toxins. Usually, whatever weight you do manage to lose on a fad diet is quickly gained back, along with a couple extra pounds for good measure. This is the classic rebound effect of yo-yo dieting, and severely impairs your metabolism, making it harder and harder to be successful the next time you go on a diet.

A natural foods diet means that you'll be eating clean wholesome foods that are devoid of chemicals, preservatives, artificial sweeteners, trans-fats and unhealthy sugars such as high fructose corn syrup. A natural foods diet allows you to safely lose excess weight, reduce or even eliminate cellulite (which is trapped and hardened toxins and lymph), eliminate an enormous amount of toxins that have been trapped deep within your cellular tissues, reset your metabolism and weight-point, and achieve greater health and well-being. You'll be flooding your body with essential vitamins and minerals from your foods, and your immune system will be kicking into high gear, so your resistance to illness and disease will greatly increase. Your mind will be sharper, you'll have more energy, and you'll notice significant and positive changes in your moods.

What Can You Eat

A natural foods diet means eating foods that are as close to nature-made as possible, and choosing organic vs. conventionally grown as much as you can. Your diet should consist of fresh, in-season fruits and vegetables, choosing canned or frozen varieties only if you can't afford or don't have access to fresh produce. If you can't afford organic produce, make sure you remove ALL peels and skins of your fruits and veggies before consuming, since this is where most of the pesticide and herbicide residues remain after harvesting. This is important, because, no amount of washing or scrubbing will fully remove the pesticide and herbicide residues that remain in conventionally grown produce. If you eat meat, only choose organic meats and wild-caught fish. Additional foods should include whole grain products and sprouted breads, raw nuts, seeds and sprouts, nut butters, and fresh or freeze-dried herbs and spices. The goal is for you to be eating mostly "living" foods, instead of lab-made foods.

Since your body will be getting supplied with the nutrients that it needs from these enzyme-rich, living foods, you will find that your level of hunger will naturally decrease. On the flip-side, when you consume a processed foods diet, chronic hunger will always be a problem because you are not feeding your body the essential nutrients it needs, and is constantly signaling you for, via hunger pangs. You can cram volumes of food into your mouth, and stuff your stomach full, but if you aren't feeding your body proper nutrition, it feels like it is "starving" and turns on your hunger switches in an attempt to get those nutrients. Simply put, hunger is a signal that your body needs nutrients, not food volume or nutritionally-void food choices. And, you body is desperately hoping that its next intake of food, will contain those nutrients that it is 'hungering' for. Fake foods will never satisfy your hunger, or your nutrient needs. Nature-made foods, on the other hand, are full of living nutrients and satisfy hunger quickly. With a natural foods diet, both hunger and cravings decrease naturally. Again, your body 'hungers' for nutrients, not food mass or volume.

Foods to Avoid

Processed foods (if it's boxed, canned or jarred, then avoid it as much as possible)

Fast foods (all)

Preservatives (shouldn't be a problem if you abstain from eating processed or fast foods)

Artificial sweeteners (replace with stevia or xylitol)

Candy, cakes and other sweets (with the exception of 70% or higher dark chocolate in moderation)

All alcohol, except for moderate wine consumption

Limit your caffeine intake to 1 cup of coffee a day, and what naturally occurs in green tea

Table salt (ONLY use REAL sea salt, which is either gray or pink in color)

The Vicious Cycle

When you consume food, your body must process it. However, your body only recognizes, and can only process natural foods, not fake lab-made foods. In fact, your body, in all its wisdom, recognizes fake foods as the toxic invaders that they are, and immediately tries to eliminate them by all means possible. However, your body can only eliminate so much fake food each time you consume it, along with the preservatives and toxins that go along with it. And, what it can't eliminate, it STORES! In order to safely store it, so you don't die of toxic overload, your body holds onto fat and tucks those toxins safely into your fat cells away from your vital organs, so you stay alive and breathing.

If you keep overloading your body with more and more preservatives and pollutants, your body then has no choice but to make more fat cells, so it can keep storing all those toxins you continue to feed it. Do you now see how the vicious cycle of eating a diet full of toxic, processed foods leads to unmanageable weight gain? This is why you NEED to constantly be detoxifying and cleansing your body, so it can eliminate those toxins and efficiently use the nutrients you feed it. When you start to clean out those toxins, you will naturally and effortlessly lose excess weight as a result.

Detoxifying and Cleansing Supplements

Along with a natural foods diet, you can support your cleansing efforts with certain supplements. Nowadays, you can readily purchase detox supplement kits online or at your local health food store, or as singular supplements, depending on your individual needs and preference. ALL people need to regularly do a liver cleanse, whether through single herbs or with a liver cleanse kit. Your liver is your body's warrior organ, and must process and eliminate all your metabolic and toxic wastes. When your liver gets congested, its function becomes greatly impaired. (I will cover liver cleansing in more detail, in the following two chapters.) Some of the common cleansing kits you can find and are recommended are: "liver cleanse kits", "kidney cleanse kits", "candida cleanse kits", "heavy metal cleanse kits", "parasite cleanse kits" and more.

Some Recommended Single Supplements

Garlic – (choose a quality brand that has a high allicin content) Garlic is nature's potent antibiotic, antifungal, antibacterial and antiviral. For continuous protection against microorganisms, and to support the elimination of toxins from the body, I recommend that garlic be taken throughout any cleanse, as well as daily, for optimal health and well-being.

Vitamin C – (2,000 - 5,000 mg daily) Vitamin C is a potent free radical scavenger antioxidant. Your body will be throwing off lots of free radicals during a cleanse, and upping your daily vitamin C intake during this time is very supportive to the process.

Milk Thistle – Milk Thistle is proven to cleanse and rejuvenate the liver, and, is another herb that I highly recommended be taken not only during a cleanse, but daily.

Ginger - If you experience any nausea or stomach discomfort while cleansing, ginger tea and capsules will help alleviate stomach cramping and nausea, and even vertigo.

Turmeric - If your body starts to throw off a lot of mucus, turmeric helps to quickly expel it. Turmeric is also a potent antiviral, antibacterial, antifungal, anti-parasitic, and has superior detoxifying properties. You can make a cup of turmeric tea, or take in capsule form.

Aloe Vera – Aloe Vera destroys pathogenic bacteria, yeast, viruses, parasites, dead cells and toxic substances, and is another highly recommended addition during any cleanse, to assist in a quicker elimination of toxins, and reducing your healing crisis symptoms.

When transitioning to a natural foods diet, you are essentially working towards a lifestyle change, and, you don't have to do it all at once. By making small changes daily, and committing to them, you will progress and keep improving your eating habits weekly and monthly. The physical, mental and emotional changes will motivate you to keep going forward. The poorer your current eating habits, the slower you should go, so you don't overwhelm your body with too many toxins to process and eliminate at any one time.

Be sure to support your healthy nutritional changes with the other detoxification methods covered in the previous chapters. Doing something as simple as taking a nightly hot bath, will help purge those toxins even faster from your body, and greatly ease the whole cleansing process for you.

CHAPTER 6 – LIVER CLEANSING: YOUR LIFE DEPENDS ON YOUR LIVER

The liver is your most important organ of detoxification, and your well-being and life literally depend on the health of your liver. Your liver functions as a powerful filtering and purification 'factory', that converts everything you eat, breathe and absorb through the skin, into life-sustaining substances. Additionally, your liver is a major blood reservoir, forming and storing red blood cells, and filtering toxins at a rate of a quart of blood per minute. It also manufactures natural antihistamines that you need to keep your body's immune responses high.

More than any other organ, the liver enables you to benefit from the foods you eat. Without the liver, digestion would be impossible, and the conversion of food into living energy nonexistent. It is your primary metabolic organ for proteins, fats and carbohydrates. The liver synthesizes and secretes bile, a substance that not only ensures proper food assimilation, but is also critical to the excretion of toxic materials from the gastrointestinal tract. Blood flows directly from the gastrointestinal tract to the liver, where it filters and neutralizes toxic substances from your food before they are distributed throughout your bloodstream. Your blood also keeps returning to the liver, processing toxins again and again through your lymph system, until they are excreted by the bile or kidneys.

Abuse and Rejuvenation

Liver congestion and exhaustion, interferes with all these above mentioned vital functions. Unfortunately, since the average American diet is high in calories, fats, sugars and alcohol, with high amounts of toxins from preservatives, chemicals, pesticides and nitrates, almost everybody has impaired liver function to one degree or another. Health problems occur after many years of abuse, when the liver is so exhausted it loses the ability to detoxify and cleanse the body of these harmful substances. Fortunately, your liver also has amazing rejuvenation powers, and can continue to function even when as many as 80% of its cells are damaged (obviously to a lesser degree of efficiency). Even more remarkable, the liver can regenerate its own damaged tissue, so that even life-threatening situations, such as cirrhosis, hepatitis, acute gallstone attacks, mononucleosis, pernicious anemia, and even major surgery or death can be averted.

One of the simplest things you can do to aid in your liver's ability to cleanse and detoxify your body, is by taking 5 deep, slow, cleansing breaths every hour. Breathing is free, and can be done by anybody, anywhere. Inhale slowly and as deep as you can (for a count of 5-10 seconds), and then exhale slowly and as fully as you can (for another count of 5-10 seconds). Deep breathing stimulates the body's lymph system, which is vital for the filtering, neutralizing and elimination of toxic substances from the body.

Benefits of Liver Cleansing

A liver cleanse is often the first vital step in any detoxification and cleansing program, and is necessary in paving a clean pathway for the body to begin to repair and heal itself. Gland function and digestion often improve right away, and, you will notice this in terms of fewer instances of swollen glands during cold and flu season, and less lower back fatigue (which is often adrenal swelling).

Additional liver cleansing benefits include seeing a reduction in stubborn weight and cellulite, especially if you currently notice unusual upper stomach distention, which is often a clear sign of a swollen liver. Both gallstone and kidney stone accretions (growth) lessen, and, drug and alcohol cravings reduce. Most women notice that PMS and other menstrual difficulties like endometriosis are far less severe, and, seemingly unrelated problems like breast and uterine fibroids, may be corrected. Male and female infertility, as well as male impotence may also show significant improvement. Inflammatory conditions like shingles flare-ups, neuritis pain and herpes outbreaks are helped, and, brown skin spots and spots before the eyes (signs that the liver is congested) begin to fade.

Signs You Need a Liver Cleanse

* Unexplained fatigue, listlessness, depression, lethargy, or lack of energy.

* Numerous allergic reactions.

* A distended stomach, even if the rest of the body is thin.

* Mental confusion, spaciness, diminished ability to focus and concentrate.

* Sluggish elimination, general constipation, possibly alternating to diarrhea.

* Food and chemical sensitivities, accompanied by poor digestion and sometimes unexplained nausea.

* PMS, headaches and other menstrual difficulties.

* Bags underneath the eyes.

* Yellowish tint and/or liver spots on the skin, poor hair texture, slow hair growth, itching skin.

* Anemia and large bruise patches indicate severe

liver exhaustion.

The truth is, everybody can always benefit from periodic liver cleansing. If your diet is poor, you have high exposure to external and internal toxins, you find yourself frequently sick, or have any of the above signs, you need to take serious consideration into doing a full-blown liver cleanse. There are many various liver cleanse protocols and liver cleanse kits to choose from, and you should choose the one that you'll most likely commit to.

Don't forget to take into account 'the healing crisis' (covered in Chapter 2), and that you will often go through a period of feeling worse before you start to feel better during your cleanse. Remember, these "ill feelings", are due to your body pulling and retrieving all those toxins from their deeply imbedded tissue spaces, and transporting them out of your body. These ill feelings are also NOT indicative that your liver cleanse is not working, or making you worse. On the contrary, it indicates that the liver cleanse is effectively doing its job, and that is to purge your body of stored-up, embedded toxins. It is especially important to drink plenty of fresh, filtered water during this time, as well as to NOT be re-depositing these same toxins into your body, by continuing to eat poorly and exposing yourself to the very same chemicals and harmful substances you are trying to rid yourself of. In other words, in addition to cleaning out your body, make sure you are also cleaning up your lifestyle habits.

CHAPTER 7 – FASTING: A JUICE VS. WATER FAST

Juicing is not new (it's been around for thousands of years), and, is a great way to jump start your detoxification efforts. Many people go on water-only regimens, and believe that it is the only true way to fast. However, a juice fast program will usually provide you with more benefits than that of water-only fasting, and without many of the drawbacks.

Preventing Muscle Loss

The right kind of juice fast will properly nourish your body, and, you won't experience the kind of muscle loss that can happen during a water-only fast. If you're a fan of the television series "Survivor", you've watched the participants wither away every week, losing large quantities of muscle mass. In essence, except for a few spoons of rice each day, they usually are on a water-only fast. Periodic juice fasting provides the body with so much concentrated nutrition, that such muscle loss would be minimal. Prepared correctly, juice fasting can provide the nutrients, amino acids and fuel that your liver requires to cleanse both itself and your body. This is an extremely important aspect of efficient and proper detoxification, because a clogged and poorly functioning liver can only cleanse and detoxify the body to a degree relevant to its own health (as covered in the previous chapter).

Antioxidants

Correctly prepared juice (meaning freshly juiced and consumed within 30 minutes of preparation) floods your body with an incredible abundance of antioxidants, which you will need to protect your liver from the enormous influx of free radicals that are released during fasting. On the other hand, water-only fasting actually decreases antioxidant stores, and does not provide your body with new incoming ones, thereby increasing your risk for oxidative damage from free radicals to the tissues and organs throughout your body.

Keep in mind that water-only fasting, and even long-term juice fasting, depletes your body of glutathione. That may not seem that important, but it really is. Glutathione is probably the most important, and the most abundant antioxidant in the body. It protects us from free-radical activity and regenerates vitamins C & E. The overworked liver is a hotbed of free-radical activity, and adequate levels of glutathione are essential for neutralizing this, to prevent the liver from sustaining significant free radical damage. Remember, the state of health of your body, is in direct relation to the state of health of your liver.

Healing

Fasting with the right kinds of raw, fresh juices increases the healing benefits of fasting. Specially prepared juices are packed-full of nutrients, phytonutrients and vital enzymes. These can supply the raw materials your body needs to repair your cells, heal your organs and protect your tissues from free radicals damage.

Juice Fasting and Weight Loss

Juice fasting is a sensible, medically sound method of fasting and can very quickly allow you to shed excess toxic fat stores that your body may be carrying - even if you're significantly overweight. In addition, you can avoid a water-only fasting trap of which many people are not even aware of. What's the trap? Water-only fasting can actually cause you to gain significant amounts of weight after the fast. After more than 24 hours or so of fasting, your body actually slows down the production of the enzyme proteins in your liver that metabolize and get rid of toxins and metabolic wastes.

That's one of the reasons why fasting with specially prepared juices is so much more sensible. Not only that, but it is also much easier to stay on a specially prepared juice fast because your body will not crave nutrition in the same way that it does during a water-only fast.

No Metabolically Induced Weight Gain

Let's go a little deeper in explaining the weight gain factor with a water-only fast. Fasting with specially prepared juices does not throw your body into a state of muscle catabolism, which is excessive muscle breakdown.

During a water-only fast, the body goes into this catabolic state and burns muscle tissue as a means of acquiring fuel. After about 2 -3 days of burning muscle, which is further broken down and converted into glucose, as the ultimate means of fuel, the body shifts to burning ketones from the breakdown of fat as fuel. So, a few days into a water-only fast, the body now begins breaking down more fat and less muscle. Sounds good right? Hold on a minute.

Long duration water fasting can result in ketosis, and the body can become quite acidic. When your body is highly acidic (also called acidosis), it accelerates free radical damage to the body, speeds your rate of aging, increases the release of your body's fat storing hormone insulin, and causes a whole host of other unwanted and dangerous health effects. Additionally, long duration water fasting slows your body's metabolic rate, and this metabolic slowdown is what can actually cause you to gain weight after the water-only fast ends, and you start to eat again.

To explain this weight gain post water fasting further, when you go on a water-only fast, mechanisms in your brain signal your body that you are starving, even if you are not. Therefore, your body goes into a survival state, trying to hold onto all of the calories it gets. In this state, you can actually eat nothing and lose only a small amount of weight.

HOWEVER, your body doesn't immediately move back out of this perceived 'starvation mode' when you start eating again, and, it may take months for your metabolic rate to recover. Thus, when you go back to eating a normal diet, you will usually gain weight rapidly, and often, you will gain even more weight than what you initially started out at. Now, if you decide to do another water-only fast, your metabolic rate, which may have never fully recovered, may cause you to continue to gain even more weight after the next water only fast is completed, causing even further harm to your body's metabolic balance and abilities.

A specially prepared juice fast can avoid these problems, and allow you to quickly rid your body of disease-causing chemicals and toxins, as well as help shed excess fat and cellulite, helping to bring your body into a much more healthy, shapely and weight-proportionate state.

Staying Energized

Many fasting programs are so physically challenging, that you can be left feeling completely wiped out, with little or no energy to function. On the contrary, a juice fast (which is loaded with the nutrients your body 'hungers' for) is designed to keep you energized enough to work, play and enjoy your usual daily activities. Juice fasting will increase both the detoxification capabilities of your body, as well as the quantity of toxic eliminations. In other words, you'll rid yourself of much more toxic waste, and, your body will be better equipped to handle this extra waste removal. Quite often during juice fasting, you may actually experience more energy during the fast instead of less, which typically tends to happen around the 3-4 day mark.

Liver Friendly

Water-only fasting can place considerable additional strain upon an already overworked liver. And, since your liver is your primary detoxification organ, you need to do all you can to support its vital function to your body, health and well-being. Juice fasting helps support the liver. On the other hand, water-only fasting usually places more strain on the liver and depletes the liver of glutathione, which is another contributing factor for the overwhelming sense of fatigue you can experience during a water-only fast.

During a water-only fast, a flood of toxins is released from cellular tissues so quickly, that the liver can become quite overwhelmed trying to keep up the process of detoxification. Such a burden is placed upon the liver at this point, that it usually requires a substantial supplementation with additional vitamins, minerals, amino acids and antioxidants. Juice fasting, on the other hand, supplies all these vitamins, minerals, amino acids and antioxidants already, lessening the overload to your liver and supporting its ability to filter, neutralize and eliminate the releasing toxic wastes.

Juice fasting is a great way to jump start your detoxification efforts, and because you'll see quick results, it can be quite motivating in helping you to transition into healthier and cleaner dietary and lifestyle habits. Juice fasting can be done for as little as one day, or as long as several weeks or more. HOWEVER, I never recommend going on a juice fast for longer than 3-5 days without first consulting with your doctor, and being under their supervision, especially if you have any current and/or major health concerns.

Additionally, juice fasting can also be supported and used in conjunction with any of the detoxification methods covered in chapters 3 and 4. A simple way of using juice fasting to maintain a healthy and clean lifestyle is to dedicate one day a week to consuming nothing but filtered water and freshly made juices.

As we continue on to Part II of this book, in the next chapter I will go over some highly beneficially juice recipes you can use to jump start your detoxification program, as well as making them a regular addition to your new, and healthier, diet and lifestyle habits.

PART 2:
STAYING CLEAN –
DETOXIFYING LIFESTYLE
PRACTICES

CHAPTER 8 – JUICE RECIPES THAT RELEASE TOXINS, STUBBORN FAT AND CELLULITE

Now that you understand a bit more about how fresh, raw juices can be a vital part of your detoxification efforts, I wanted to include some

The following, are highly recommended juice therapies that will kick-start weight loss, including those stubborn last 10-15 pounds. These juicing remedies are also recommended for keeping your body in proper acid - alkaline balance, as well as maintaining optimal digestive health. You may use them at any time, and ideally you'll want to regularly include juicing into your healthy nutritional lifestyle.

If you have never consumed fresh, raw juices before, you may wish to wait until the weekend to try them, for they will help speed things along in your digestive system, and you'll be spending a bit extra time in the restroom, so plan accordingly. Once your body gets used to fresh, raw juices, you can easily consume them at any time. Any diarrhea you may experience in the beginning, is you body purging toxic waste (healing crisis), which is what you want, so welcome these extra trips to the bathroom.

Juicing Recipes

ONLY use organic produce! Otherwise, you're defeating the purpose of detoxification. Eating whole, or juiced, commercial produce, only serves, to reintroduce MORE toxins into your body, via chemical pesticide and herbicide residues.

Lymphatic Detox Drink

3 green apples (cored and quartered)

3 large celery stalks (stems and leaves removed)

1 small cucumber (rough chopped)

6 leaves kale

1/2 of a lemon (peeled and quartered)

1 (1 inch) piece fresh ginger (peeled)

Run all ingredients through your juicer, and, drink immediately.

Metabolism Makeover Drink

2 apples, any variety (cored and quartered)

1 large grapefruit, very thinly peeled (you want as much of the white pithy part, between the peel and the flesh of the fruit, to remain)

2 large celery stalks (ends and leaves trimmed)

5-6 fresh mint leaves

Run all ingredients through your juicer, and, drink immediately.

Whole Body Cleansing 'Cocktail'

2 large lemons (peeled and quartered)

1 large apple (cored and quartered)

1 large pear (cored and quartered)

1 large garlic clove

¼ inch fresh ginger root (peeled and rough chopped)

1 cup hot water

1-2 teaspoons of raw honey (do NOT use processed honey!)

Dissolve the raw honey, into the 1 cup of hot water. (Use an extra large mug to do this, since you'll be adding extra ingredients.) Run the rest of the ingredients through your juicer, and pour into your hot honey water. Stir to blend, and, drink immediately.

Liver Cleansing Elixir

2 large cabbage leaves

1 large garlic clove

1 C chopped cauliflower florets (make sure you use the florets, not the stems)

½ C chopped broccoli florets (again, make sure you use the florets, not the stems)

1 large red variety apple (cored and quartered)

½ C chopped fresh parsley

Run all ingredients through your juicer, and, drink immediately.

Fat and Cellulite Dissolver Drink

3 large carrots

2 large, ripe tomatoes

1 cucumber (rough chopped)

Run all ingredients through your juicer, and, drink immediately. If you can take a little 'heat', this juice tastes incredibly good, with a few dashes of your favorite hot sauce. And, the capsaicin in the hot sauce, will add even more fat, and cellulite-melting benefits to this drink.

It is vitally important to remember, that you will NOT get these same detoxifying and cleansing benefits from consuming bottled or canned juices, which have been pasteurized and processed. This processing destroys all the 'live' enzymes, as well as most of the micronutrients contained in the fruits and vegetables, which is where most of the healing benefits come from. Quality juicers are much more affordable these days, and you can easily find one in your price range. Adding a juicer to your kitchen is one of the best things you can do to support a health and clean lifestyle.

CHAPTER 9 – TOXIN TRAPPING FOOD

If your schedule doesn't accommodate the ability to do a juice fast, or full detoxification regimen, but, you still want to cleanse and detoxify your body, and perhaps even jump-start your weight loss efforts, then a great way to do that, is to start include some toxin-trapping foods into your daily diet. Nothing fancy or expensive, just some of Mother Nature's finest detoxifying foods to help you purge those toxins and waste matter from your body.

Detoxifying Foods

Avocados

A single, medium-sized avocado contains up to 30 grams of Omega-9 essential fatty acids, which is a unique type of fat that prevents hunger pangs and cravings. In addition, Omega-9's also are essential in helping the liver break down fat more efficiently. But wait, there's so much more avocado goodness. Just half of an avocado contains a whopping 8 grams of fiber, plus a healthy dose of monounsaturated fatty acids (MUFA's). MUFA's are healthy fats that increase production of the metabolism-boosting hormone adiponectin. Studies show that consuming just one avocado daily, can help you lose up to 10 pounds in 2 months, without counting calories. Even better, avocado eaters lose an average of 56% more belly fat than non-avocado eaters.

Free-Range Omega-3 Rich Eggs

Nearly 100 chemical reactions must occur in the liver in order to flush out fat-soluble toxins. In order to do its job, the liver needs a steady supply of taurine, cysteine and methionine, and just 2 eggs daily can deliver all the key amounts of these three important amino acids.

Citrus Fruit

Eating just 1/2 cup of fresh citrus fruit daily, blocks the absorption of diet-sabotaging saturated fats before they can be shuttled into your body's fat cells. Researchers give credit to the soluble fiber found in citrus fruit (pectin), as well as its toxin-neutralizing antioxidants, including hesperidin, d-limonene and glucarate. Eating half of a grapefruit, or one small orange 30 minutes before each meal, offers amazing fat blocking, toxin flushing and calorie reducing benefits.

Flaxseed

Flaxseed contains 800 times more lignans

(compounds that help the liver metabolize toxins), than any other plant, providing superior detoxifying benefits. In addition, flaxseed's soluble fiber and Omega-3 content cut blood sugar and insulin surges by as much as 30%, which significantly helps to prevent fatigue, eliminate brain fog, squash hunger and even lift blue moods.

Raspberries

Each single cup serving of these yummy, sweet berries, provide a whopping 8 grams of fiber as well as fat-fighting ketones. Rasberries also contain phenolic compounds, which have been shown to trigger a biochemical process in which fat cells release stored fatty acids. This benefit alone, has led pharmaceutical companies to try and isolate ketones for inclusion in weight loss supplements. However, it is just as easy, and more delicious, to get your fat-burning ketones directly from the source. So, load those fresh raspberries on your yogurt, oatmeal and other healthy dishes, as well as enjoy them all on their own.

Beans

Just a single serving of legumes provides a whopping 15 grams or more of dietary fiber (50% of your RDA), as well as 15 grams of appetite-suppressing protein. This combination of fiber and protein has been proven to help people flush out toxins and fat (especially belly fat) two times faster than non-bean eaters.

Metabolism Boosting Spices

If you want to rev-up your cleansing and detoxification efforts even more, while at the same time giving a natural boost to your metabolism, then you'll also want to regularly add the following spices to your dishes, for even more toxin flushing, calorie and fat burning benefits.

Ginger - This tasty Asian spice can turbo-charge your metabolism by 20% for up to 3 hours after consumption. Simply slice or grate it into your favorite stir-fries, salads and veggie dishes, and, fresh ginger is great in smoothies and muddled up together with some fresh mint leaves, and added to a glass with some crushed ice and sparkling mineral water.

Cayenne Pepper - Just a pinch of this fiery spice added to your hummus, soups, chili and other dishes will boost your fat burn by 10% for up to 3 hours after eating.

Mustard – Most people are surprised to learn that this tangy condiment favorite revs metabolism by an amazing 25%. Darker mustards seem to increase your metabolism slightly more than lighter varieties, but just about any mustard variety is great at stoking your fat-burning furnace.

Cinnamon - Cinnamon contributes to your fat loss and metabolism boosting efforts by its amazing ability to lower and keep blood sugar levels stable, as well as curb your cravings. In addition, it even helps lower cholesterol levels. Aim for getting 1/2 -

1 teaspoon of this spice daily, or you can take a cinnamon capsule with each meal.

Cleaning-up your diet is always a critical component in whole body detoxification, and in achieving and maintaining good health and a proper, healthy weight. While doing a full nutritional cleansing regimen a couple times a year is recommended and ideal, some people can be too intimidated by this, and prefer a more gradual approach to detoxification and cleaning up their diet. Adding toxin-trapping foods to your daily diet, while at the same time throwing out the junk food and processed foods, is a great way of doing just that.

CHAPTER 10 – WHOLE BODY DETOXIFICATION AND CLEANSING THROUGH SKIN BRUSHING

When referencing the organs of the human body, most people immediately think of their liver, lungs, kidneys, etc. But, did you know, that your body's largest organ, is actually your skin. On the average size adult, the skin covers approximately 3000 square inches, and, makes-up about 15% of your total body weight. Our skin acts as a barrier, helps to regulate body temperature, expels waste and secretion, and, is rugged, flexible and practically waterproof. Our skin protects against trauma, and is slightly acidic, to ward off and help prevent bacteria, from entering our body. Our skin is so vital, and provides so many functions, yet, it is possibly one of the most overlooked, and neglected, parts of our body.

Questions:

Q. What organ is responsible for a full 1/4th of your body's detoxification processes?

Q. What organ eliminates a full 2 lbs of acidic waste from your body every day?

Q. What is one of the most important elimination organs in your body?

Q. When the blood is full of toxic materials, what organ will reflect back these affects?

Q. What organ is the last to receive nutrients in the body, yet the first, to show signs of imbalance or deficiency?

The Answer to All of These Questions Is:

Your Skin

Vigilance, in keeping your skin healthy, plays an integral part in maintaining balanced, whole-body health and well-being. How can you assist in keeping your skin healthy? Well, one of the most important things you can do, in keeping your skin healthy, is to put into practice, the ancient and still used art, of SKIN BRUSHING.

Many various cultures have used the art of Skin Brushing for centuries, including the Greeks, Japanese and American Indians. Some formerly used methods of skin brushing, included using the backs of large spoons and ladles, dried corn cobs, and even sand to accomplish this task. In fact, the Texas Rangers still use the sand method, to regularly skin brush, for vitality and health today. Today, however, the most commonly used method of skin brushing, involves using a natural fiber skin brush to accomplish the task.

Benefits of Skin Brushing:

* **Colon Cleansing** - Dry skin brushing stimulates the lymph canals, to drain toxic mucoid matter into the colon, which significantly helps to flush, and purify, your entire system. In fact, after several consecutive days of skin brushing, you might notice gelatinous mucoid material in your stools. This gelatinous mucoid material is actually old, stagnant waste that has been accumulating in your body. Good riddens!

* **Aids Lymphedema** - Skin brushing literally moves the lymph material containing large proteins and particulate matter, that cannot be transported in any other way, back into the circulatory system. If these proteins stayed in our systems, outside of our blood vessels, it would then start to attract other fluids to these locations, and, pretty soon, we would find ourselves with painful, swollen joints and limbs. And, once severe enough, eventually we'd actually be leaking fluid, right out of our skin. This condition is called lymphedema, and, is why all health and wellness programs always involve some type of exercise and/or body work. It is because the flow of blood, oxygen and lymph, is absolutely essential for our health and well-being.

NOTE: Dry skin brushing can be of vital necessity for invalids, and those recovering from accidents, are in a coma, wheelchair bound, or have limited mobility.

* **Muscle Toning** - Skin brushing stimulates nerve endings, which in turn cause individual muscle fibers to activate and move. This also helps to redistribute fat deposits, and, again, is of great benefit to those who are immobile, or who have limited mobility.

* **Cellulite Control** - Cellulite is a non-scientific term, defined as hardened, toxic deposits of subcutaneous fat material, and fibrous tissue, that are not able to be readily eliminated, and, which often cause a dimpling effect on the overlying skin. Skin brushing aids cellulite, by stimulating the lymph system to rid our body of these accumulated, toxic materials, and flush them from our body through our normal excretory channels. All detoxification, starts first and foremost with the lymph system, so, skin brushing is a vital key in ridding and preventing cellulite. To target your cellulite areas, use deep, circular brushing movements for at least 10 minutes, twice per day. Always, follow-up your skin brushing with a warm shower or bath, ending with a cool rinse, and drinking at least 1-2 glasses of purified water.

** If you want to "kick-it-up-a-notch", and, do what they do in expensive body spas, follow-up each cellulite, dry skin brushing session, with a salt or sugar rub, before taking a shower or bath. This will help to further release stubborn toxins that are deeply embedded within your body tissues, and, it also stimulates quick, and healthy, skin cell renewal. If you are frustrated and tired of dealing with your cellulite, make a commitment to do a 5-10 minutes dry skin brush, followed by a salt/sugar scrub on a daily basis before your shower, and, you are guaranteed to see fabulous results.

* **Whole Body Detox** - Whether you are on a cleansing diet, or not, your body requires the constant intake of vital nutrients, and, the constant output of toxic waste. And, skin brushing, helps to accomplish both of these critical needs. Skin brushing dilates your pores, allowing toxic waste material to easily exit the body, while simultaneously allowing necessary nutrients to enter. Regular skin brushing readily prevents a "log jam" effect, which can result in dandruff, eczema, psoriasis, red skin patches, acne, boils, constipation, herpes outbreaks, cellulite formation, and more. Additionally, when lymph flow is not stimulated and becomes backed-up, this can cause a dangerous increase in one's blood pressure, which is just one of the many reasons why, in addition to skin brushing, walking is so beneficial to one's health. Walking can be done almost anywhere, at your own, individual pace, and, is one of the best, and easiest, ways to stimulate your body's lymph system. Furthermore, stimulating your body's

lymph system is important for strengthening your immune system. A strong, well-functioning immune system is necessary for killing, and fighting off, harmful bacteria, viruses, and other microbes.

* **Skin Health** - Dry skin brushing sheds dead skin cells, allows for maximum nutrient absorption into body tissues, improves skin texture, increases the rate of healthy skin cell renewal, tightens skin (this is great while on a weight loss program, or, to tighten loose, sagging skin), and so much more. Regular skin brushing will literally cause your skin to have a healthy glow, from head to toe. You will experience increased energy, regular digestion, rid yourself of troublesome skin problems, and, keep yourself looking younger than your biological years.

The Art of Skin Brushing

The art of skin brushing is quite simple, yet, incredibly therapeutic. It involves taking a dry, natural fiber body brush, and brushing your naked skin with it, using various, directional stroking movements, and, with various depths of intensity. It takes a mere 5 minutes or less, unless you are doing the cellulite removal protocol, and ideally, should be done at least once per day. The best time to perform skin brushing is just before taking a bath, shower or sauna. Skin brushing will open up the pores, remove dead skin cells, and, stimulate the body's lymph system and removal of toxic debris.

The heat of a bath, shower or sauna will accelerate, and heighten, this cleansing process, as well as immediately increase the circulation of oxygen, blood and nutrients throughout your body.

Rules of Skin Brushing

While there is no need to do any specific type of brush strokes when skin brushing, there are however, a few basic rules you need to follow.

1. Always brush in the direction of your heart. It doesn't matter if you are going from head-to-toe, or toe-to-foot, as long as you remember this vital rule. Using strokes that go away from the heart, puts extra pressure on the valves in your veins and lymph vessels, which can potentially cause ruptured vessels and varicose veins. So, remember, to always brush stroke in the direction of your heart.

2. Only brush your skin when it's dry. Brushing your skin when it's wet will not have the same effect, and benefits, and, you'll just be stretching, and causing potential damage, to your skin.

3. Only use a natural-fiber skin brush. Synthetic skin brushes, will only serve in scratching your skin. If you want to achieve scratching, you can just run through your nearest section of dense trees and shrubs. Kidding of course, but you get the message.

4. Use appropriate stroke depth. This is easy to remember, because your body will react

accordingly, and give you immediate "feedback', if you're doing it wrong. Use lighter brush strokes on thinner and more sensitive skin areas, and, go a little deeper on thicker and less sensitive areas. NEVER skin brush your nipples, genital area, varicose veins, open wounds, cuts, new scar tissue, bruises, or face. That should cover all the obvious, but please, don't try to override common sense.

5. Regularly wash your skin brush. Once a week, wash your skin brush with a natural liquid soap (I use castile soap) and hot water, and allow your brush to fully air dry before using again.

To skin brush, your starting point can either be at your feet, or at your hands. The goal is to brush as much skin as you can comfortably reach, making long, even-pressured strokes in the direction of your heart, and brushing 3-5 times in each area, before moving on to the next area. So, for example, brush your left arm from wrist to elbow on all sides, 3-5 strokes on each side. Then, move on to brush from your elbow to your armpit, covering all sides, again, making 3-5 strokes on each side. Do all parts of your body this way, and, remember to always brush in the direction of your heart, and use lighter brush strokes on any sensitive areas. (Also, remember to avoid brushing the caution areas, listed above.) When just starting to skin brush, you may find your skin to be extra sensitive to the process. This especially tends to be the case, in people who lead sedentary lifestyles, and, those with heavily congested lymph systems. In either case, start off with lighter brush strokes, and, try skin brushing every other day, until your body becomes acclimated.

The benefits of skin brushing are many, and, the effort minimal. Just a few quick minutes, before your daily shower or bath, is all it takes. Make skin brushing, a part of your daily grooming regimen, and you'll very quickly start to experience the many wonderful detoxification benefits this ancient health practice has to offer. Watch your cellulite disappear, loose skin will tighten and tone, your body will have a natural rosy glow, and, skin disruptions will often self-resolve. And, yes, you really will begin to look years younger than your biological age!

CHAPTER 11 – FLUSH TOXINS WITH THESE DETOXIFYING BATH RECIPES

In today's world, no matter how healthy your lifestyle is, it is virtually impossible, to completely avoid being exposed to chemicals, toxins and other pollutants. And, it goes without saying, that all chemicals, toxins and pollutants, are harmful to your body and health. Therefore, adding to your list of detoxifying lifestyle practices, one which is also arguably one of the most pleasant of detoxifying and cleansing methods, is a good old fashion, soak in the tub.

Even a plain bath, in nothing more than hot water, is beneficial. However, it's been proven, that even just a short 20 minute soak, in a detoxifying bath, can successfully flush out loads of chemicals, toxins and other pollutants from our body. These contaminants are constantly entering, and accumulating, in our bodies. And, if these contaminants are not regularly purged from our body tissues, they will quickly become major contributing factors to a host of unwanted health consequences, such as stress, weight gain, mood disturbances, skin disruptions, cellulite, digestive complaints, and more. And, if left unchecked, will eventually lead to even more serious health conditions. (Hopefully, you're getting this repetitive message by now.)

A hot bath dilates and opens skin pores, allowing the release of toxins from our waste-carrying lymph channels, located just beneath the skin. Adding simple and easy to get ingredients to your regular bath can turn it into a powerful, detoxifying soak, that you can use as often as you like. (Note: Those with heart conditions of any kind, as well as women, who are pregnant, should only use bath therapy under the care and guidance of their health care provider.)

Easy Detox Bath Recipes

<u>Salt and Soda Combo</u> - The pH of bathwater makes a huge difference in how the body eliminates toxins. As a by-product of metabolism, as well as the constant accumulation of toxins, our body produces acidic waste which greatly impairs the flow of lymph. Unlike our heart and other body systems, our lymph system has no pumping mechanism, and relies on both physical movement, and sweating, to move and purge these trapped toxins and waste products. When this doesn't happen regularly, a backlog of waste and toxins occurs, causing cellular inflammation, and leads to body aches, pain, unexplained fatigue, skin conditions, the inability to lose weight and mental fogginess, just to name some of the many health consequences.

Fortunately, soaking in alkaline water will help rebalance your body's internal pH, and diminish, or even eliminate, many of these unwanted health consequences. A salt-and-soda detox bath, can relieve cellular inflammation and its related symptoms by almost 50%, and is especially beneficial for those who experience constant all-over body aches, arthritis and gout sufferers, lupus, fibromyalgia, chronic fatigue, and other auto-immune disorders. This bath requires 2 cups of either dead sea salt or kosher salt, and 2 cups of baking soda. Add the salt and soda to your bath water when the tub is approximately 2/3's full, and stir the water to fully dissolve before entering tub. You can double this amount if you have a large tub.

Seaweed - A seaweed bath is beneficial for everyone, but especially for those who've suddenly gained weight, can't lose weight regardless of a good diet and regular exercise program, and those with cellulite. Health experts have long known that the minerals in seaweed have a strong and powerful ionic charge that draws toxins out of bodily tissues. Additionally, while pulling toxins out of the body, at the same time, seaweed also pulls in vital nutrients that haven't been able to get into the body's cell tissue, due to the cells being clogged with toxic wastes. This important 'garbage-out and nutrients-in' activity is vital, and helps release trapped fat as well as diminishes cellulite.

Seaweed varieties, especially bladder wrack and laminaria, are rich in iodine, a vital element that optimizes thyroid gland function, thus speeding up metabolism and revving up production of the important fat burning enzyme lipase. And, good news for aging skin, seaweed also contains alginates, polymers that enhance skin suppleness and counteracts sagging skin. You can buy seaweed bath soaks at your local health food store and through reputable vendors online, the latter of which, is a much cheaper option. You can even purchase pure seaweed varieties in bulk on eBay, for even bigger savings. Mermaid costume optional!

Epsom Salt - Don't underestimate the powerful healing effects of regular Epsom salt. Soaking in hot water infused with Epsom salts (magnesium sulfate) boosts blood levels of the ever important mineral magnesium, by as much as 35% in just 1 week. Magnesium is a critical mineral that too many people are deficient in. If you suffer from muscle tightness, stiffness, spasms, aches and pains, then buying Epsom salt in bulk and adding it to a hot bath 3 times a week, will bring magical relief to your discomfort. The magnesium in Epsom salt will also bring much wanted relief to those who find themselves in a chronic state of tension, stress and anxiety.

The human body requires magnesium to manufacture the 2 enzymes quinone reductase, and glutathione S-transferase, both of which assist in neutralizing and eliminating chemical toxins. Being deficient in magnesium, puts a significant damper on your body's detoxification abilities. Magnesium also plays a critical role in regulating nerve and muscle activity, to help shield the body against the ravages and dangerous cumulative effects of stress. Add 2-4 cups of pure Epsom salt to a hot bath several times a week, and see for yourself the incredible difference it makes. Epsom salt baths can often turn even the most "bath-shy" guy, into a tub lover.

Most people can enjoy these detoxifying baths as often as they like. The exception would be for those who suffer from any type of heart condition, epilepsy, narcolepsy, and pregnant women, all of whom, should only use bath therapy under the guidance and care of their health care provider.

CHAPTER 12 – HOW EXERCISE DETOXIFIES THE BODY

The importance of regular, moderate exercise for the human body cannot be overstated. The human body is kinetic, and is designed for movement. Chronic lack of movement, results in the stagnation and accumulation of metabolic wastes and toxins, diminished circulation, and reduced oxygenation in the body. This then creates the conditions, and sets the stage, that can lead to weight gain, skin disruptions and disorders, mood imbalances, system imbalance, disease and cancer. The human body needs to move everyday, and moderate, regular physical activity should never be an exception, but rather a rule.

With all of today's modern conveniences, as well as the hectic pace in which we live our lives these days, most Americans are quite deficient in the amount of exercise and/or physical activity they get. Lack of regular physical activity, along with a poor diet and other bad lifestyle habits, makes for a lifetime of sickness and ill health, including obesity. On the other hand, regular moderate physical activity keeps our weight in balance, our muscles flexible and toned, our bones strong, our immune system running strong, our mood balanced, our skin clear, and then, a magical reverse of circumstance happens. Instead of exercise being the exception and occasional concern, it is disease and ill health that have now become the exception and occasional concern.

Exercise and the Circulation of Blood, Lymph and Oxygen

Regular, moderate exercise truly has an amazing and powerful rejuvenating effect on the entire body. It stimulates the circulation of blood, lymph and oxygen throughout the body, and these substances are vital in the distribution and trafficking of nutrients to our cells, as well as the removal of waste products. As you know by now, anytime blood or lymph distribution is slowed down, toxic substances cannot be adequately removed, and our cells literally choke on their own metabolic waste. Additionally, anytime oxygen distribution is slowed down, and your organs cannot get sufficient quantities, they start to deteriorate. Organ function is then compromised further and further, until finally, disease and unwanted health conditions take hold. Regular, moderate exercise ensures that proper and adequate amounts of blood, lymph and oxygen are always circulating throughout the body, helping to keep all of its components healthy and balanced.

Exercise and Detoxification

Exercise is a natural detoxification process, and works to continuously remove harmful toxins, pollutants, and other substances from your body, before they can take residence within the cells of your organs, blood and fatty tissues. It also keeps your immune defenses purring along at optimal function, thus warding off colds, flu and other infections. In fact, after a bout of exercise, white blood cells remain elevated for up to 2 hours afterward, during which time they are busy cleansing and detoxifying the body. Building up a sweat is another important part of exercise, as well as to the detoxification process of our body. One of the major functions of your skin is that of elimination. For those who suffer from gout or any form of arthritis, your body has a build-up of harmful uric acid. When you perspire through physical activity, the acidic waste product uric acid is excreted through the dilated pores of our skin, making it an important function in the removal of toxins, and the healing of your condition.

Again, the importance or regular physical activity and exercise cannot be overstated, but remember, exercise alone will not help you if you continuously subject yourself to poisons such as processed foods, fast foods, smoking, over-indulgence of alcohol, drugs (street, over-the-counter or prescription) and chemically-laden personal and household products. No matter what your current health condition, there is always some type of physical activity you can do, even if it's limited. So, get moving, and make sure your body is engaged in regular daily movement, and regular moderate exercise, as part of your healthy, whole body detoxification regimen.

CHAPTER 13 - MERCURY FILLINGS: A CONSTANT SOURCE OF POISONING

While we have the ability to detoxify most of our body tissues from harmful toxic wastes, there is one area of concern, in which our ability to cleanse and detoxify is almost completely disabled, and avoidance is the absolute best form of preventative detoxification. And, that area of concern is most likely in your mouth right now.

Metal dental ware is a constant source of poisoning and allergic reaction to the human body, especially, when dental ware is exposed, and in contact with, milk and other dairy products. All metal corrodes with time, especially in the mouth, where there is a high concentration of air and moisture. Among other harmful metals, amalgam fillings contain the extremely toxic mercury. Mercury actually makes up to 50% of the filling! Mercury vapors are constantly being off-gassed in the mouth and transported into the lungs through inhalation, before then entering the digestive system while eating and drinking. When the mercury vapors finally enter the blood and lymph, they can cause considerable and cumulative damage within the body, most especially, the nervous system. In recent years, researchers have produced unique videos that show the constant mercury vapor escaping from the mouths of people with metal fillings in their teeth. Most of us have amalgam fillings, and, are being exposed to mercury poisoning every day. I strongly urge you to look this up online, and see for yourself, the powerfully negative effects mercury fillings are causing to your body, every single day.

Other Countries Say "NO" To This Toxic Metal

In Germany, a federal law passed back in the mid-1990's, prohibits dentists from giving mercury fillings to their patients. For the same reason, most of North European countries have limited the use of amalgam, and Sweden, Spain, Austria and Denmark, amongst many others, have outright banned the use of this toxic product in the year 2000. The amalgam compounds are so toxic in fact, that dentists are instructed to not touch it with their bare hands, and amalgam must be stored in special tightly sealed containers. If it is so dangerous to even touch amalgam, it suffices to believe, that it certainly must be even more dangerous to keep in one's mouth for the remainder of one's lifetime, or to get it injected into the blood with a flu vaccine!

The Absolutely Alarming Health Consequences

It is noteworthy to point out, that patients with Multiple Sclerosis (MS) and Alzheimer's disease have up to 10 times the normal amounts of mercury in their brains. Post-mortem studies show that the mercury level in some organs is directly proportional to the number of amalgam fillings in a diseased person. And the most vulnerable of all to mercury poisoning, seems to be the developing fetus in pregnant women. A fetus accumulates more mercury than even the mother does, and in amounts directly proportional to the number of the soon-to-be mother's amalgam fillings. This is the reason why pregnant women should avoid tuna and other mercury-containing fish during pregnancy, and while nursing. You might want to re-read the last few sentences again if you are pregnant, or know someone who is pregnant, to fully grasp how dangerous mercury is.

The gradual, continuous release of mercury and other toxic metals into the body via metal fillings, particularly affects the liver, kidneys, lungs and brain. Additionally, cadium which is used to produce the pink color in dentures, is 5 times as toxic as lead! It does not take much of this metal to raise one's blood pressure to abnormal levels, yet, how many people are aware that they might be developing a heart condition as a result of the dental fillings in their mouth?

Thallium, which is also found in mercury amalgam fillings, is known to cause leg pain and paraplegia.

It also affects the nervous system, skin and cardiovascular system. ALL wheelchair patients who have been tested for metal poisoning, test positive for thallium! That's one heck of a common denominator. Many people in fact, who became wheelchair bound for several years after they received metal fillings, completely recovered once all metal had been removed from their mouth. Thallium is lethal at a dose of only .5 - 1.0 gram. Who approves this stuff to be safe for human use?! The FDA, the AMA, and all those other so-called consumer safety oversight agencies, do.

Additionally, other metals contained in dental fillings are known for their cancer-causing effects. These include nickel (used in gold crowns, braces and children's crowns) and chromium (which is extremely carcinogenic). All metals corrode (including gold, silver and platinum) and the body absorbs it. It is proven, that women with breast cancer have accumulated large amounts of dissolved metals in their breasts. When the mouth is cleared of all metals, metal residues will eventually also leave the breast tissues and the metal-caused cysts will shrink and disappear by themselves. Chronic yeast infections also often quickly improve after removal of metal fillings. Some men report complete relief of prostate problems, after metal filling removal, as well as relief from chronic nose and sinus congestion.

Unfortunately, porcelain can be toxic too. It is made of aluminum oxide, along with other metals added. The body's immune system naturally responds to the presence of toxic metals in the body, and eventually develops allergic reactions which may show up as a sinus condition, ringing in the ears, enlarged neck and glands, bloating, enlarged spleen, arthritic symptoms, headaches and migraines, eye diseases, and more serious consequences such as paralysis or heart disease.

Composites

Although metal toxicity may not be the only cause for these aforementioned conditions, replacing all metal fillings with composites, greatly assists your immune system in its ability to detoxify and protect your body against ill health and disease. A composite filling is one that is primarily non-metallic. There are a large variety of materials used in composite fillings, but, some metals may be present. Ordinary composites are not suitable for large cavities. Whenever used for large cavities, they tend to last no more than 5 - 6 years. Indirect composites, on the other hand, can be placed in large cavities. They can even be used in place of gold crowns. They look like a real tooth, and last as long as gold. If selected properly, indirect composites are quite non-allergenic and non-toxic. They are fairly new and can be as expensive as gold fillings, but, they can save you a whole lot of health trouble and money in the long-term. Since many dentists don't know how to place them properly, you may need to do a bit of research to find an experienced mercury-free dentist who also works with indirect composites. The fillings should be replaced cautiously and gradually, 1 or 2 at a time. It is also best, not to replace metal fillings more often than once every 2 months.

Preventing Heavy Metal Toxicity

Prior to Filling Replacement

If you decide to replace your amalgam fillings, make certain that your dentist provides for protection (through a special plastic device) against the inhalation and absorption of the generated amalgam dust. Otherwise, you may end up suffering severe migraines, memory loss, weakening of eyesight, and more. Before attempting to have any larger fillings removed, you may need to take selenium (if possible in ionic form) for 1 -2 months prior to replacement.

Everyday Prevention

Eat more foods that contain vitamin C, as well as more red-colored fruits and vegetables. Use cilantro and green leafy vegetables in every main meal. These are natural chelating foods that help flush mercury and other metal deposits from the body. Drinking several cups of Pau d'Arco tea per day (or taking capsules) for 2 weeks on, and then 2 weeks off in rotation, may also greatly assist you in the detoxification of the blood, liver and kidneys. A kidney cleanse is also highly beneficial in assisting the removal of metals from your system, as well as preventing injury from any released metals.

CHAPTER 14 – PURIFY YOUR HOME'S AIR ENVIRONMENT WITH PLANTS

Because we spend so much time indoors in today's world, keeping the interior environment of our home detoxified and clean, is every bit as important, as keeping our body detoxified and clean. Houseplants are pretty to look at, but, you need to give them more credit than just being beautiful. Mother Nature is smart, and has imparted amazing and powerful cleansing and detoxification abilities and properties to the many plants and flowers in the botanical kingdom. Plants silently and diligently work hard to purify the air in our living spaces, as well as aid us in maintaining good health. Plants increase oxygen in our living spaces, remove toxic chemical off-gasses, help you sleep, relieve allergies and headaches, and even reduce mold.

So, if you're looking for just the right houseplants to both beautify and purify your home, check out these plant marvels below, and choose the species that best suits your family's needs.

Banish Mold with English Ivy

Musty basements, damp laundry rooms, and anywhere moisture collects, are breeding grounds for mold - AND excellent spots to place English Ivy. Researchers have found that when the vines were brought into a room, 60% of airborne mold VANISHED!

Care Tips: Ivy is shade and cold-tolerant, so it can be put practically anywhere. Even in a drafty room or dark hallway. Keep soil damp, and mist regularly.

Relieve Your Allergies with Rubber Plants

Rubber plants have a high humidity content, which draws dust and allergens to them effortlessly like a magnet. Dust and allergens stick to the plant's leaves, instead of lingering in the air and irritating you.

Care Tips: Rubber plants are practically worry-free. They only need low light, cool temperatures and a drink of water when the soil is dry, which is about once a week.

DID YOU KNOW....That just looking at plants is a proven stress-reducer. Plus, plant leaves give off negative ions, airborne molecules, that are research proven to boost your mood and help alleviate depression.

Fight Asthma with Boston Ferns

Nothing beats Boston ferns, for removing harmful formaldehyde from the air. Formaldehyde is a toxin commonly found in furniture, clothes and carpeting, that can irritate your eyes, nose and throat, and, is a common trigger of asthma symptoms.

Care Tips: Boston ferns love shaded light, and plenty of moisture. Mist them frequently, or put them in a humid environment, such as the bathroom or kitchen.

Banish Headaches with Orchids

What do paints, cigarette smoke, ammonia, dry-cleaning chemicals, plastics and chemicals all have in common? They're all headache-inducing culprits that are commonly found in many homes. While you should first be striving to be removing these toxic offenders, you can also clear away their harmful off-gasses found in your home's air, by placing some lovely orchids throughout your living spaces.

Care Tips: Although they look delicate, orchids don't require any special care. Just provide them with some medium light, cooler temperatures, and avoid overwatering. Just once a week should do it.

Freshen-Up Your Bathroom with Peace Lilies

Peace lilies are one of the best plants available, for absorbing common chemical vapors like acetone (found in nail polish remover), and alcohol (found in hair products and household cleansers).

Care Tips: Peace lilies will "tell you" when they need watering, by drooping their leaves. Once you give your lilies some water, they will perk right back up again. And, don't worry if your bathroom isn't sun-drenched, as Peace lilies prefer indirect light, and can thrive even under fluorescent lighting.

HOW MANY PLANTS DO YOU NEED TO PURIFY THE AIR?....You'll need 1-2 full sized plants, to filter the air in a 10x10 room. The more, the better.

Purify the Air and Clear Your Head with Golden Pothos

Golden pothos are highly adept at absorbing toxic benzene. Benzene is found in plastics, many cleaning products, and tobacco smoke. Benzene causes drowsiness and dizziness.

Care Tips: Be careful, to not overwater. Let the soil completely dry out in-between waterings. Once or twice a year, be sure to clip back the leaves to keep them full.

Superior Air Purifier with Bamboo Plants

Bamboo palms are superior for removing the worst 3 household toxins - Benzene, Formaldehyde and TCE. Bamboo also pumps much-needed moisture into the air, especially during the cool weather months, when humidity levels are typically low.

Care Tips: Bamboo prefer bright, filtered light. Also, allow the top layer of soil to dry out in-between waterings.

Purify Air after Household Projects with Dracaena

Put some Janet Craig Dracaena in a room or work area, after painting or doing some furniture repair. Dracaena gobbles up odors and the toxin TCE found in paints, lacquers, varnishes and adhesives.

Care Tips: Dracaena prefer bright light, but, don't put them in direct sun. Water thoroughly, but do allow the soil to fully dry in-between waterings. Also, mist its leaves often, and wipe them with a damp cloth.

Oxygenate Household Air with Snake Plants

Snake plants work dutifully overnight to lower levels of carbon dioxide in the air. This keeps oxygen levels higher during the day, resulting in much better air quality, which allows you to think clearer and be more productive.

Care Tips: Snake plants are practically indestructible. They thrive in any kind of light, from semi-sun to shade, and, only need watering when the soil is dry to the touch.

Sleep Like a Baby with Bromeliads

Some plants actually give off more oxygen during

the night, and Bromeliads are one of them. Unlike most plants, they give off high levels of oxygen during the night instead of during the daytime hours, helping you breathe easier during the evening hours and while you sleep. Therefore, you'll definitely want to place one of these tropical beauties in your bedroom.

Care Tips: Bromeliads like to soak up lots of light and warmth, so be sure to place them in a sunny spot during the day, and then move them close to your bed when you go to sleep. When watering, you'll want to pour the water directly over the center of the rosette in the middle of the plant.

So, beautify, purify and detoxify your home, by filling it up with some of Mother Nature's botanical wonders. And, as you can see by the easy care tips of most of these purifying and health-boosting plants, you don't need to be a seasoned "Green Thumb" to make them thrive.

CHAPTER 15 – 15 DIY, CHEMICAL-FREE GREEN CLEANING RECIPES

Keeping your family safe from chemical overload should not be such a daunting task, yet we are bombarded by what seems to be, a plethora of toxic, chemically-laden cleaning products in our markets and stores.

Fortunately, the good news is, there are easy, cheap and highly effective homemade cleaning recipes that you can make in your own home, using easy to find, cheap ingredients. There is no need to expose your family to the harmful effects of all those potent and toxic chemicals in household cleaners. Chemicals that are proven to cause everything from headaches, to skin irritation, learning disabilities, auto-immune disorders, cancers, neurological problems, and on and on, so, why would you want to clean with this stuff, and expose your family to these toxic dangers?

Go to your local dollar store or discount store, and purchase some large spray bottles, for mixing, storing, and using your homemade, household cleaners. Be sure to make a waterproof label for each bottle, so you always know what's in them. You still want to keep your homemade cleaning products stored safely away from children and pets. Also, use common sense. Only use these homemade household cleaners for their intended purpose, and, if you're allergic to any of the listed ingredients, then don't use them. And, speaking of allergies, ALL humans are allergic to chemical household cleaners.

HOMEMADE WINDOW CLEANER

Add 1 cup of white vinegar and 1 cup of rubbing alcohol to a large spray bottle, and then fill the rest of the bottle with water. Use to spray on mirrors, windows, and chrome, to get a chemical-free cleaning and shine. Additionally, try swapping out paper towels with newspaper, or a lint-free towel you dedicate to using with the window cleaner, and wash periodically. Solution will keep indefinitely.

HOMEMADE ALL PURPOSE BATHROOM CLEANER

Mix the following ingredients in a large spray bottle: 1 cup baking soda; 1/2 cup dish liquid soap; 1/2 cup water; 1/4 cup white vinegar. Using a small funnel will help you to combine the ingredients in this mixture. (double the ingredients, for larger spray bottles) This mixture is good for cutting through soap scum and killing mildew. Solution can be safely used on tile and porcelain surfaces. Shake spray bottle well before each use.

HOMEMADE BLEACH

Mix the following in an empty, rinsed out plastic gallon container. (such as a milk, juice or water container) 1 cup hydrogen peroxide (3% over the counter); 3 tablespoons of lemon juice; and 10 cups of water. Shake gently before each use. Solution will last 3 months, so be sure to date your container label. Also, do NOT rinse out and re-use a commercial bleach container.

HOMEMADE OVEN CLEANER

I recommend repurposing an old plastic food container that has been cleaned out, for storing this effective oven cleaning paste. Combine 1 cup white vinegar; 1 cup borax; and 1 cup baking soda. This cleaning paste cuts through most greasy oven messes with ease, but, it can also be left to sit on older, hard-to-remove oven messes overnight, and cleaned off the next day. Apply and use this paste with a scouring pad, or scrubbing brush. Rinse off freshly cleaned oven surfaces with a wet rag, soaked and wrung out in hot or warm water.

HOMEMADE CARPET CLEANER

Mix the following in a spray bottle: 1 tablespoon white vinegar; 1 tablespoon ammonia; 4 cups cold water. Shake mixture, spray on stain, and let soak for a few minutes. Dab (don't rub) the stained area, and repeat until stain is lifted. You can also make this solution in larger quantities, and use in a carpet steam cleaner.

HOMEMADE CARPET STAIN REMOVER

Mix the following in a spray bottle: 1/4 cup liquid dish soap (good brands are 'Seventh Generation', 'Earth Friendly', 'GreenShield'); 1/3 cup water; 1/8 cup white vinegar. Shake bottle well, spray onto stain, and allow solution to sit for a few minutes, before dabbing area with a clean, wet rag.

HOMEMADE CARPET FRESHENER

In a non-metallic container, mix together 1 cup baking soda with 1/2 cup cornstarch and 3 drops of your favorite essential oil (lemon, pine, lavender, etc.). Mix well, and then sprinkle this mixture evenly onto your desired carpet areas. Allow to sit overnight, and vacuum up powder the next day. This carpet mixture helps to pull pet and other odors from your carpet, and the essential oil imparts a nice fresh scent. This DIY carpet freshener is easy to make in large quantities, and then stored in a shaker-dispenser bottle, such as is used for Parmesan cheese and pepper flakes.

HOMEMADE ALL-PURPOSE CLEANER

Mix 4 tablespoons of baking soda with 4 cups warm water in a large spray bottle, and shake well. This easy to make solution, can be safely used on tile, stainless steel, vinyl, ceramic and glass surfaces throughout the house, for cleaning, gentle scouring and deodorizing purposes. (Do NOT use more baking soda than the recipe calls for, otherwise you'll need to do an additional water only rinse.)

HOMEMADE LEATHER CLEANER

Now you can clean your own leather surfaced items (car seats, jackets, etc.) with the following mixture of 1/4 cup olive oil and 1 teaspoon lemon oil (not lemon juice). Buff your leather items with this mixture to get rid of dirt, as well as get a nice glossy shine.

HOMEMADE WOOD FURNITURE CLEANER

Whisk together 1/8 cup lemon juice with 1/4 cup olive oil, in a small, non-metallic bowl. Apply solution to wooden surfaces with a soft, clean cloth. This mixture helps to darken scratches, as well as give your wood furniture an effective green cleaning.

HOMEMADE VINYL CLEANER

This recipe is great for cleaning outdoor patio furniture, as well as vinyl couches and chairs. Mix together 1/4 cup white vinegar, 1/4 cup vegetable oil, and 2 cup of water in a spray bottle. Shake well before each use, spray onto desired vinyl surface, and rub with a soft, clean cloth.

HOMEMADE VINYL FLOOR CLEANER

Here is a great recipe for keeping your no-wax floors clean. In your mop bucket, combine 1 tablespoon of liquid dish soap (such as 'Seventh Generation', 'GreenShield', 'Earth Friendly') with 1/2 cup white vinegar to each 1 gallon of hot water, and then mop as usual. This solution really helps to easily lift dirt and grease right up off your vinyl floors.

HOMEMADE HARDWOOD FLOOR CLEANER

This recipe not only cleans your hardwood floors, but also helps to cover scratches at the same time. In your mop bucket, combine 8 black tea bags with 4 tablespoons of olive oil for each 1 gallon of hot water, and then mop as usual. This will clean, help cover scratches and give your floors a nice shine.

HOMEMADE LIQUID FABRIC SOFTENER

In a plastic container with a tight fitting lid, combine 1 cup of white vinegar, 2 cups baking soda, and 4 cups of water, and then shake well. Add 1/2 cup of this mixture to your wash RINSE cycle, for fresh, static-free clothes. (tip: rinse out and use a gallon size juice or water container)

HOMEMADE CLEANER FOR PAINTED WALLS

This super simple mixture will help take those wall smudges off without ruining your walls. In a spray bottle, combine 1/ 2cup of white vinegar with 32 ounces of water. Shake, spray onto desired areas, and wipe with a soft, wet sponge or cloth.

You really can achieve superior cleaning results, without endangering your family with all those chemicals in store-bought cleaning products. Not only are you protecting your family's health, you are also protecting your family's budget, because all these recipes are so cheap to make.

Other helpful tips:

* Even though these are chemical-free mixtures, some people have sensitive skin, so wearing gloves is always a good idea when cleaning.

* You can always cut the recipes in half to make a smaller amount, or double to make larger amounts.

* Always be sure to label your mixing bottles, and put some clear masking tape on top of the label, so it stays waterproof and readable.

* Remember to always store all household cleaning products safely out of reach from children and pets.

As part of your overall detoxification and clean living lifestyle, you can now clean your home, without the worry of harmful and toxic fumes and residues lurking everywhere for your family to be exposed to, potentially causing a multitude of health problems.

CONCLUSION:

So, there you have it. An easy to follow, get clean – live clean lifestyle program that anyone can do, starting today, for a healthier state of well-being. Since most of these methods are low cost solutions, finances should never be an obstacle in your detoxification efforts. Once you embark on your cleansing practices, and your health and well-being improve, your results will be a powerful motivating factor to continue living a cleaner lifestyle. Not just for you, but for all those who bear witness to your healthy transformation.

Here's to a cleaner, healthier you!

Gina

ADDITIONAL BOOKS BY AUTHOR

- Natural Cures: 200 All Natural Fruit & Veggie Remedies for Weight Loss, Health and Beauty

- Easy Vegetarian Cooking: 100 – 5 Ingredients or Less, Easy & Delicious Vegetarian Recipes

- Natural Foods: 100-5- Ingredients or Less, Raw Food Recipes for Every Meal Occasion

- Easy Vegetarian Cooking: 75 Delicious Vegetarian Casserole Recipes

- Easy Vegetarian Cooking: 75 Delicious Vegetarian Soup and Stew Recipes

- The Veggie Goddess Vegetarian Cookbook Collection: Volumes 1-4

- Easy Vegan Cooking: 100 Easy and Delicious Vegan Recipes

- Vegan Cooking: 50 Delectable Vegan Dessert Recipes

- Holiday Vegan Recipes: Holiday Menu Planning for Halloween through New Years

- The Veggie Goddess Vegan Cookbook Collection: Volumes 1-3

- Healthy Living: How to Purify Your Body in a Polluted World

ABOUT THE AUTHOR

Gina 'The Veggie Goddess' Matthews, resides in sunny Phoenix, Arizona, and has been a lover of animals, nature, gardening, natural living and, of course, vegetarian cuisine since childhood. 'The Veggie Goddess' strongly encourages home gardening, supporting your local farmers and organic food co-ops, preserving the well-being of Mother Earth, and supporting and protecting animal rights.

http://www.theveggiegoddess.com

http://www.facebook.com/theveggiegoddess

http://www.pinterest.com/veggiegoddess

http://www.cafepress.com/VeggieGoddessMarketplace